GOD
IS BIGGER THAN
COVID

GOD IS BIGGER THAN COVID

My Covid-19 Experience

FRANCES L. DEANES
Maurice Dean

Superior Publishing LLC.

CONTENTS

DEDICATION POEM

Dedication Poem
To those of you who fought and fought to the end,
even though we don't know each other, I feel like we are
friends.
To those of you that lost loved ones, and you thought
they died alone,
I promise they had angels beside them to escort them
safely home.
We don't understand why we made it and others lost the
fight.
Maybe God was giving us a chance, a chance to get something right.
We know we cannot question Him; Just accept His undy-
ing Love.
The only One that has answers is our Father up above.
Wear your mask, wash your hands and stand 6 ft apart.
Because when you hear that you are positive, It will pierce
you through your heart.
2020 brought us sorrow, misery and pain

and some people really prospered and had great financial gain.

2020 tested our faith and Sometimes
it was really hard, but in all these trials and tribulation it brought me closer to God.

So wear your mask, wash your hands and stay 6 ft apart.

Because the person's life you save maybe the closest to your heart.

CHAPTER 1

When Covid Came to Mississippi

When Covid Came to MS
I Met Covid

The first closest case we heard about was, Memphis, TN. That was too close too home. Honestly we began to panic some. Shelton had family that lived in Memphis. We watched as well as prayed, hoping and praying that whatever this was making people fall dead like this would go away.

It got closer, then it invaded Mississippi, came in with luggage! I mean after all, we knew it wouldn't be long because people were moving around too much. Then it hit home for us. It was a MIND thing, we started fussing, and begging and pleading to my children and my grandchildren about how serious Corona Virus was. They thought we had gone off the deep edge.

I knew that I was watching it every day all day! I was keeping up with the counts, because they weren't. I knew that my husband and I were older and one of my daughters had underlying conditions and as a parent our job was to protect her. I began to feel as if they weren't paying any attention to what my husband and I were saying. We sang the song constantly, "Stay home, Wear your mask, don't go to nobody house, wash your hands, don't take the mask off, don't eat out, and the list kept growing.

I must admit that it was affecting my mind because it was something different, something no one really knew about, not even the doctors and it seemed like my family wasn't paying it any mind.

My husband and I made the hardest decision not to go to church. We both grew up in church. I am a Sunday school teacher and he is a Deacon. We had pretty much decided that we would have church in our home. We had two children that were preachers, a daughter that was a keyboard player and another son that played the bass, so that's what we did, we had church at home! We even went Facebook Live and shared it with the world. Church at home was good. The Holy Spirit moved in the house, just as it did in the church. We shouted in the house, just like we did in the church. The atmosphere in the house shifted just like it did in the church. We were content even though there is no other place like the house of the Lord.

Shep decided that he would stop going to the barbershop and his hair began to grow out. I wasn't big on beauty shops are anything, so I hang around the house all day watching CNN, day in and day out.

We had seen how make-shift morgues were being erected in New York and other states, no place to keep the dead, Covid had taken over. I was operating now on FULL

FEAR and still preaching to my children and my grand-children. "Wear your masks, stay at home!" My husband began to threaten to put my grandchildren out because they were moving around too much, wouldn't listen. Fear had about frozen us. We had almost just stop going out, we would just send at what we needed most of the time. The house had gotten to be closing us in even though we had much room. And Shep's hair was getting longer and longer.

It was Just A Matter of Time.....

I have a big family outside of my husband and children. I have nine

other sisters and brothers we couldn't get together any more. No more gatherings. We couldn't see each other, fear was setting in all around us. We would talk on the phone, keeping check on each other and we learned how depression was setting in on us. This virus had came and separated my family. This was nothing but that old devil, separating families.

And then, it was just a matter of time, some of my brothers had gotten it, and my heart was about to explode from fear of what would happen to them. My prayer life was deeper now, because there was no other option. We were all calling each other, it just felt like the breath had been snatched out of our bodies. We were listening to hear something but there was nothing to hear.

I remember in one of the home worship services, I had a chance to just release, because worrying about my brother had taken a toll on me, he lived so close to me, but yet it was still so far away, because of Covid. He was my go to person and just hearing him on the phone, his voice was weak, it wasn't him. I could only pray more. My heart just shook on the inside of me. "Lord pull him through this. And thank God, he got better.

And I thought about when my brother John preached at my dad's funeral, and he said, when Roger died; we cried, Mu-dear died; we cried; Moses died; we cried again and now here we are at daddy's funeral and we are crying again. I wasn't thinking about my brothers dying but we cried when the first one got sick and now... the other one had gotten it and he we are crying and worrying again. Lord have mercy this is just like being on a roller coaster and there is nothing fun about it.

One of my brothers that lived across the road from me called and said, when he found out that one of our other brothers had it, he just wept like a baby. He said he couldn't stop his tears. He told the Lord, "Please don't take my brother." He said the Lord always answers his prayers, and thank God He does, because that brother got better. He still has complications, but he is back up and preaching.

God is an awesome God. He might have allowed this Covid to come in, but He is getting the glory out of our lives. We couldn't be more grateful the Lord was pulling the family through. I Met Covid.

CHAPTER 2

Mentally, Physically & Spiritually

Mentally, Physically and Spiritually

You would think after fearing this corona virus the way that I did, after preaching to my family, after taking the necessary precautions. Even after stalking my daughter's church LIVE to see if she had on her mask, to see if the Pastor and members had on their masks and making sure my son and his family were wearing their masks at his church. Then after my daughter's had left their jobs for safety reasons to keep from contracting the virus. After we've sat sanitizer, disinfectant spray at the door for my immediate family ins and outs, after Shep had stop going everywhere but except to see about the cows alone on his tractor, and the sacrifice of allowing his hair to grow out like this, we still ended up coming face to face with Covid.

My daughter had informed us on Messenger that she had it. My heart dropped, not my Amy, not my beautiful baby, not my rider, my love lol! (*Of course I'm typing this for mom so I can say all the nice things I want to about myself lol)* Lord I knew if Amy had it, there was no way I didn't because she's always around me. We had just been together riding to Starkville, sitting in the house laughing and talking, cooking and eating, the things we do every day and now, she is on Messenger in the family group saying, "POSITIVE"

Lord what now? But of course, immediately my throat started feeling itchy.

I started to have this little dry cough, my sinus was draining and then there was this thumping in my ear. Headaches started coming, I had it.

CHAPTER 3

Mentally

So, I went and got tested, POSITIVE! My Mind went to work! I was being reminded of how many people that had already died. The numbers that I saw everyday on CNN and now on the local news station was terrifying. The count was growing every day.

The News comes on and all you can see is that little ugly corona ball with the horns sticking out of it. And now this little demonic thing has invaded my and my daughter's body. Then I'm reminded how the people looked on ventilators, Lord I was about to be stiff. The hospitals are running out of beds and now I have it! Then there it goes, Jackson, MS was buying refrigerated trailers to keep their dead. Mercy Lord, and now I have Covid!

I'm being reminded of all the people that I knew that had died, some were my cousins and some of our friends. People I had known all of my life! I'm no better than them, they contracted Covid and died. Lord now I have it too.

Seeing the people on the machines everyday was stuck in my mind, lying there hooked up all alone, no loved ones, dying by themselves on face time, husbands and wives dying within hours of each other. And here I am POSITIVE.

With all the information I already had stored in my mind how did I let it get up on me? Now I'm face to face with Covid-19, as a matter of fact, this deadly virus is now in my body. All the time I had been worrying about it coming into my house now it's in my body. I had been worried about my daughter with underlying conditions catching it and being alone in a hospital and can't remember her medicines, and can't remember when she was supposed to take them now I have it and I am in the house with her.

By this time Shep's hair had gotten even longer, I think he was always more worried about it than me with good reason, he had underlying conditions.

My family depended on me and the only ONE I had to depend on now was GOD. But God is a Healer, I had to get myself together and stay focus, because this virus had a mind of its own. I had to do the work and have faith that God would bring me through.

No wonder the Lord wanted us in the marvelous light, because nights were the worst, not just the physical but the mental state this virus puts you in. I would wake up hoping for daylight. The nights were so long and the time would only be 12:10 A.M. it was so dark and so lonely. I would try to fall asleep but wake up again. The time would only be a little after 3:00 A.M. still dark.

There is just something about the darkness. I feared every night, thinking that I wouldn't make it to daylight.

My mind would say, "If you could just make it until the morning."

Even though daylight was better, there was a change in the neighborhood. The word was out that we had it, some of my daughters, me and my husband, so we noticed the change in the hospitality. People would ride by and not wave, well not even look out at the house anymore. We were used to people almost coming to a stop in front of the house looking and being nosy, but now they would speed through looking straight ahead. My neighbors would go inside if we came outside and shut all the doors. I felt like a leper. Lol! Lord have mercy! Even though I would come down the hallway saying, "I'm unclean, and I'm unclean as the lepers did in the bible, but to actually be treated that way was mind blowing. It dealt with my mind as well. But I knew that they were afraid. Even the dog knew something, when I would take my evening walk to get vitamin D that I needed, he began to bark at me. This virus was demonic! It carried a spirit that couldn't be denied. It was a thief!

The thief, the bible says, "Comes to steal, kill and destroy" This virus tried to steal my mind, kill my body and destroy my faith in God. But in that same verse Jesus said, "I COME that they may have life and have it full or more abundantly!" Hallelujah.

I thank the Lord for keeping my mind.

CHAPTER 4

Physically

After the early signs of this virus my body started to ache, my whole body. It seemed like the virus had taken control over me. My head hurt so bad, I almost wanted to take it off for a minute and sit on the dresser. My ears were constantly thumping, like someone moving furniture around or something. Lord my nose was dry but I could smell that Covid. It was an awful smell. But then after a while, Covid took my sense of smell away. I noticed that I was spraying a lot of bleach and disinfectant but I still couldn't smell anything. And then my body had gotten so weak. Covid took the taste out of my mouth. I had an itch in my throat that made me cough and it seemed like I couldn't cough it out, the cough was so bad it made my whole body shake. My chest was sore and my lungs didn't want to breathe. My stomach was upset, and now that word is and understatement, because I was truly upset with this virus called Covid. My hands seemed to be upset as well because they ached sooo bad! My fingers, my hips, my legs, all the way down to my toes were just aching, it was so bad until I could only close my eyes.

Don't even mention my back and legs, they were wobbly it seemed as if they could go at any time.

I could see my sisters and brothers calling me but I couldn't answer them and even when I did I felt like I couldn't talk and breathe at the same time, and my coughing was so bad talking was a no-no anyway.

It was sneaky, that Covid would make you feel like you were okay and then it would snatch it back the next minute. It was so unpredictable. Most of the time, I feared hitting the floor. It was just the devil toying with me just made me unstable.

I tried to sit up most days but I would be too tired, all I wanted to do was lay down. After getting worse, I decided to move back into my own bed, because when I found out I was positive, I didn't want to expose him as well. But now it was obvious that Shep had Covid too. So I got at the foot of the bed and let him have the head. I then fixed us a little medicine table next to the bed for the midnight hour aches and pains. I was just trying to make things easier on us.

CHAPTER 5

Spiritually

After coming home as a positive Covid 19 patient, my granddaughters went to get tested. They were both negative and moved out the same day. I didn't want to see them go, but I knew it was for the best being 21 and 16. Shep had tested negative the day before and here I am positive. I couldn't stay in the room with him even though his test said NEGATIVE I knew he was POSITIVE but yet and still I moved into my granddaughter's room. The world I lived in was getting lonelier and lonelier, but I remembered, the Lord will never leave us nor forsake us.

That first night was one of the longest loneliest nights of all the long lonely nights. I was in a foreign land in my granddaughter's room. I moved a few baby shoes around, which it seemed like it must've been decoration or something for the headboard. I wanted to see out those blinds so I moved baby shoe, after baby shoe. I just had to see the light come through the blind early that morning.

I listened to gospel music on my phone and dosed off to sleep. A bad headache woke me about 2:00 A.M. took some extra strength Tylenol that worked for a while, and then woke up to day light. Glory to God! Just to see the daylight, knowing, that I have a virus in my body that has killed so many, everyday that I opened my eyes was just another blessing.

My daughter Angelica was put on quarantine from her job, so she and Tawana were here. I feared for Tawana, this had been my biggest fear since Covid came to town, was Tawana getting it, with all her underlying conditions. So we all wore masks in the house and kept our distance. It was a lonely place, no laughter, loud talking, it just seemed desolate. When I was up walking around everyone else would be confined to their rooms. When they would be up, Shep and I would be in our rooms.

Shelton was beginning to get pretty sick. He had started having chills, chest aches and coughing a lot. I was feeling so tired and helpless, then Angelica became our little nurse. She pumped us with vitamins, pain pills, juice and breakfast.

My daughter Amy is usually the one who takes care of all of us but she was at home with covid as well, again I felt helpless. But I tried to stay focused on getting better so I could take care of them. Tawana stayed in her room most of the time so it wasn't hard staying distant from her, but Angelica on the other hand, I had to keep running her out of my room, telling her to keep her mask on in the house. I think she was afraid that I was going to die. But through it all, God was still holding us up. And we were still holding on. The devil was working but God was in control.

When I felt okay, I would take long walks during the day around the yard for exercise trying to keep moving around but it was the nights that were so horrible. Lying in my granddaughter's bed, I was soaking wet, the covers were soaked, and I was hurting so bad I couldn't move. My back was weak, my fingers, head, legs and even my TOES were aching. Even though my medicine was right next to me, I couldn't reach them. I forced my hands to reach up toward heaven and I begin to say, "Hallelujah, Hallelujah Hallelujah!" And then the Lord gave me the strength to turn over to get my medicine, that extra strength Tylenol and that Dollar General blue cough and mucus. I think I took three whole bottles during my ordeal.

Thinking back to a moment, when I was lying in so much pain and I wasn't even able to reach and get my medicine off the table, all I could say was, "Lord Help Me!" And out of nowhere at that very moment, Shelton came in and popped the light on and asked me where were the pain pills?" he needed some too. Lord Jesus, all I could say was, "Thank You Jesus!"

It's funny now, but we often say, He may not come when you want Him but He's always on time! Glory to God He was right on time, I was lying there in my sweat, hurting and couldn't move myself, weak with no strength and the Lord sent my husband in the room.

We went through some aches, pains, sweats, diarrhea, weakness, coughing but through it all I never stopped praying or lost my faith in God. And Glory to God, He never left us nor did He forsake us.

Whatever the devil planned, he didn't succeed. He only pushed me closer to the Lord.

CHAPTER 6

The Long Hauler's Effect

I don't know about anyone else, but my Covid experience has changed a lot of things in my life.

For one, my tolerance is very low, I get agitated very fast and lot of times I can see my cell phone ringing and I just can't even answer it, I don't want to talk. I think I was traumatized and I'm just not dealing with it well. The last days of my quarantine, I would just walk off, just go some place and just cry my eyes out. I thought about I could have lost my family members and my husband and even my own life. I began to think about who was going to take care of Tawana and her kids, the hurt and pain my family would have endured.

Even though I knew that if I had died I would have been with the Lord. And even though I know that life goes on when I'm gone, while in my sickness I had time to think about all of those things.

The world now seems different, and the things that I

once thought was important, isn't really that important anymore.

The enemy came to steal and kill but God! I can say boldly that the Lord is my light and my salvation, and He is definitely the strength of my life.

And I know if it hadn't been for the Lord on my side, even though me and my family are no better than anyone else, we would have perished. It was God's grace and mercy.

In my close of this book, I just want to say, "Social distance yourself, wear your mask and wash your hands.

Even though God spared my life I don't question His will. So many people have died with this and I know some of them were way better than me. I thank God for showing me that He is BIGGER than COVID.

The Lord never said that there wouldn't be storms in our lives, but He will get in the storm with us.

As I write at this moment, on the news in Los Angeles, California, they are telling people if someone called or even if they look like they are going to die don't bring them to the hospital, there is no room, no oxygen tanks and they can't even resuscitate them.

No room huh? This makes me think about when there was no room for JESUS. And He had to be placed in a manger in a barn because there was no room. They gave the lowest place to the Highest King.

This is what has happened, there is no room in our lives for God any more, we've pushed HIM out. And now we can't do anything BUT DEPEND ON GOD to rescue us to save us, to sustain us.

I thank God that we made it through, even though still now we are dealing with some lingering effects. God is still able.

CHAPTER 7

Medication List

Faith and Prayer:
they work together then I began to take the following
medications.

Vitamin C
Vitamin D
Zinc
Tylenol Extra Strength capsules
Dollar General Cough & Mucus (blue liquid)
Herbal Tea
Ginger Tea

I tried to take Black Seed Oil, but it tasted like oil off a
dead body YUCK! I just couldn't do that one. And
again, the many prayers of the people that prayed for me
and my family.

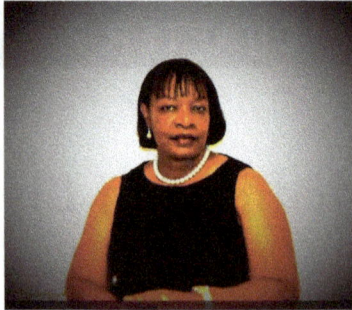

Author Frances L. Deanes
Picture by Amy Deanes

A life long resident of Abbott, MS, Frances Deanes, is the proud daughter of the late George and Emma Lou Nance Bowen. She gives credit to her parents for bringing her up in a God fearing home with 12 other sisters and brothers.

Author Frances Deanes is married to Shelton Deanes, a loving husband and they share eight beautiful children, nine beautiful grandchildren and five and a half awesome great grandchildren.

Frances Deanes loves teaching Sunday School and singing in the choir at Palo Alto MB Church also located in Abbott, MS.

She gives God all the glory, honor and praise for the things that she's endured in her life that prepared her for the Covid-19 experience.

www.ingramcontent.com/pod-product-compliance
Lightning Source LLC
Chambersburg PA
CBHW071036050426
42335CB00050B/1795